AF685648

Optimize Your Life Series

Cozy Fasting

Healthy & Hygge Habits During the Holiday Season

STEPHANIE EWING

Copyright © 2023 by Stephanie Ewing.

All rights reserved. No part of this book may be used or reproduced in any form without written permission except in the case of brief quotations in critical articles or reviews.

Printed in the United States of America.

For more information, or to book an event, contact :
StephanieEwingAuthor@gmail.com or visit
http://www.stephanieewingauthor.com

Acknowledgements

Oh I am so excited you are reading this book! Two of my favorite things are combined into one wonderful habit this holiday season. Cozy Fasting brings you health and a sense of calm this winter. Enjoy!

Cozy Fasting was written for your education. It is not a replacement for professional medical advice. If you decide to try any form of fasting, talk with a licensed health professional about your specific situation and then make your individually informed decision. The author is not qualified to provide medical, financial or psychological advice or services. The author does not guarantee results and is not paid for recommending books, apps or products in this book.

Contents

Introduction

Winter's here, the season when snowflakes dance from the heavens and we all turn into human burritos wrapped in fuzzy blankets. A time when nature drapes itself in a blanket of frost, and the world slows down just a touch. Birds fly south, animals huddle together for warmth, and the mere thought of emerging from under the blankets before the crack of dawn seems like a cruel joke played by our alarm clock.

For this winter season, I want you to consider a practice that brings a wealth of health benefits and will make your cozy indulgences seem even sweeter. When many are stuffing their stomachs at holiday parties and overindulging on eggnog, we're going to be talking about - not eating. We'll delve into fasting, a practice shown to improve metabolism, enhance brain health, and even extend lifespan according to studies. It's a journey through both the science and the art of mindful eating and not eating.

Think of it less as denying yourself and more like giving yourself a different kind of treat. It's not just about ditching the Christmas cookies because just one won’t hurt . . . It's about finding those moments of clear-headedness even when it's foggy outside.

And, when the fasting window closes, I've got you covered with recipes that'll make your post-fast meals feel like a hug in a bowl. Pull up a soft chair by the fireplace, and let's set the stage for a winter of warmth, comfort, and mindful eating. Who knows? By the time the first buds of spring appear, you might just have a whole new relationship with your plate and your palate. You will have figured out the secrets to happy fasting and be in the midst of enjoying all the healthy side effects.

Chapter 1

Why Fasting?

Winter's charm can be a double-edged sword. Twinkling lights beckon us to a whirlwind of parties, and our plates become battlegrounds for decadent meals, creamy desserts and sugar cookie armies. Our calendars? So filled with events it resembles a paint splattered canvas, and the familiar chime of the cash register leaves our wallets thinner with each jingle.

But imagine steering this winter in a different direction. Picture this: instead of that redundant holiday party, you're cocooned in a chunky knit blanket with spiced tea warming your hands. Bypass the mall mayhem and spend an afternoon crafting homemade gifts or penning heartfelt letters. Consider giving the constant grazing a break, sprinkling in days of mindful fasting to make festive feasts all the more delightful.

What if, instead of a frenzied dash from one event to another, we took time for snowy walks, savoring the muted world beneath our feet? Rekindle the joy of board games by candlelight or get lost in a book by the fireside, soaking in those 'hygge' vibes that prioritize comfort over chaos.

This winter let's seize the reins and reclaim our time. Let's focus on the warmth of connections, not just the warmth of our ovens. By consciously choosing to step back from excess, we open up space for what truly nourishes our hearts and souls: quiet moments of reflection, laughter-filled evenings with loved ones, and the deep satisfaction of enjoying the season in its purest, coziest form.

Things to Let Go of This Winter:
The Calorie Carousel: Ditch the urge to sample everything in sight. Balance fasting with feasting and relish each morsel. In all aspects of our lives, many of us have forgotten a very important truth. Too much of a good thing can end up being very harmful to our health. Working together, we can reclaim our health and enjoy those rare indulgences even more.

Calendar Chaos: Simplify December. Choose meaningful moments over back-to-back activities. How many Christmas parties do we really need to attend? Create a cozy spot in your home, sip on some tea and read a good book. You will feel less stress and more hygge.

Wallet Woes: Gift-giving doesn't necessitate emptying your bank account. Embrace value-driven gifting that emphasizes experiences. Think about this: the next time you are given a Christmas mug filled with yummy hot cocoa – do you judge the gift giver? Do you tell them you already have too many coffee mugs? Nope, you accept the gift and cherish the thought behind it. Crochet a kitchen towel, paint a set of coasters, or make a yummy treat – remember the gifts you give don't need to cost a lot of money to be cherished.

Things to Embrace This Season:
Mindfulness: Find delight in the season's subtle moments - whether it's a family chuckle or the soft glow of festive lights. Set aside time each morning to journal about things that make you feel grateful and bring those feelings with you throughout your day. Reflect on your journal when you feel your stress level rise and take deep breaths. Imagine smelling pine trees as you inhale and blowing out a candle as you exhale.

Putting Loved Ones First: Prioritize genuine connections. Cherish stories shared by the fireplace and revel in memory-making. Watch a movie together, work on a craft or play a game with Christmas songs on while sipping on a warm beverage – these things will fill yours and your loved one's emotional buckets and help you be more resilient.

One of the most beloved holiday traditions in my family involves baking sugar cookies. Not just any sugar cookies, these are painted sugar cookies. We make the cookie dough ahead of time and refrigerate it. Then we get out our food-grade paint brushes and create our "paint" in holiday colors using 1 egg yolk, water and food coloring. Then we cut out fun shapes and paint our cookies before we bake them. The paint turns out shiny and the cookies are beautiful and delicious. Before my sister-in-law joined the family – we just painted, now with her artistic side, we have more fun! Snowmen dressed in their swimsuits, obviously headed for the beach, camouflaged reindeer trying to get out of pulling the sleigh and stars featuring bursts of color make our cookie trays much more fun! I am sure Santa gets a laugh from the cookies we leave for him on Christmas Eve too.

Handmade and Customized: Ditch mass-produced for personalized. A simple, well-thought-out gift, like your homemade caramel-apple butter or a unique snowman family drawing (While my SIL can do this by hand, I need to give props to Midjourney for the AI assist!), speaks volumes. One year, my mom made meals in a jar for us for Christmas. We had a variety of soups, casseroles and even desserts all layered in mason jars and ready for us to enjoy. She even cut out holiday-inspired fabric and wrapped the top of each jar with ribbon.

Fasting & Feasting: Explore a balanced approach to indulgence. Feast with gratitude and fast with purpose. Using the tips in this guide, you will be able to fast with warm, yummy drinks and enjoy your holiday treats even while losing unwanted weight. I think the energy you will feel while fasting may surprise you too!

As winter envelops us, let's champion simplicity and intentionality. Let’s celebrate a season that shines not because of the glitter and glare but because of its genuine warmth, comfort, and the small joys often overshadowed yet profoundly impactful.

Do It Yourself

Smoked Sea Salt

If you haven't tried smoked sea salt - you are in for a treat. Smoked salt can be purchased in the store and there are many to choose from. You can use smoked salt on anything, however I think it adds a delicious flavor to deviled eggs, french fries and even dark chocolate or caramels. If you own a traeger or other smoker grill then this recipe is for you.

Smoked Sea Salt Instructions:

1 pound sea salt
3 hours on the smoker
1 aluminum pan
Optional: splatter guard fine mesh

Add the sea salt to the bottom of an aluminum pan, or place it evenly spread on the splatter shield and rest that on the pan. Smoke on low temp, about 170 degrees for 3 hours, stirring every 30 minutes. Remove from the smoker and let cool. Place in small decorative sealed jars and gift with a salt spoon and beautiful label for a truly delicious and unique gift!

Below are the instructions to make smoked sea salt in your oven. You will need to purchase liquid smoke, and parchment paper.

Oven Smoked Sea Salt Instructions:

Preheat your oven to 200 degrees. Just fill the container you are using for the smoked sea salt as the measuring tool and pour that into the bowl. Make sure to add an extra tablespoon to ensure it's full. Then pour the liquid smoke (up to 1 tablespoon per heaping cup of sea salt) into the salt a few drops at a time and stir until combined. Repeat this process a few drops at a time to make sure the salt doesn't start dissolving.

Line a cookie sheet with parchment paper and pour the salt onto the sheet and spread it out. Place in the oven for 10 minutes. Use a spatula or spoon to give the salt a mix to make sure it doesn't form clumps. Put it back in the oven for 5 more minutes. Allow to cool for a few minutes before adding to your container.

Use the smoked salt as a dry rub on meats, for fajitas, or rim your margarita glass for a unique drink. Truly you can use smoked salt as a replacement for regular salt in any dish you choose - it is up to your tastes.

Chapter 2

The Art of Fasting

Fasting, with its deep-rooted history, feels like a cherished heirloom passed down through humanity's seasons. Fasting stands as a timeless tradition. Beyond sculpting our physical form, fasting also soothes our restless minds, much like the beauty of a quiet winter night.

Its benefits extend beyond physical health; studies have shown that fasting can enhance brain function and mental clarity. For instance, research in the 'New England Journal of Medicine' highlights that fasting can improve cognitive performance and stress resistance, echoing the tranquility of a serene winter night.

In today's bustling world, our thoughts flutter about like the first snowflakes of winter, frequently settling on the idea of our next meal. Can you believe that nearly 30% of our mental landscape is painted with thoughts of food? Venturing into fasting feels like stepping into a snug, quiet cabin. This introspective journey opens up a pristine, tranquil space where we can engage and reflect.

Fasting at its core is the decision to abstain from eating for a length of time. I encourage you, as you begin this journey, to be flexible and use the advice in this guide to assist you in making your decision to fast. Fasting, when done with this warm guidance, can be as comforting as a hug from a loved one.

Fasting is Embedded in our Biology

Journey back to an era without instant meal deliveries or buzzing kitchen gadgets. A stark, yet comforting simplicity where our ancestors, instead of awaiting a delivery, played a game with nature for their sustenance. And yes, nature often had the upper hand. But, in those gaps of finding food, rather than surrendering to fatigue, our forebears found renewed energy.

Skipping a meal or two not only honed their hunting strategies but also sharpened their minds. The benefits were holistic: from clearer cognitive pathways to an internal cellular cleanup. Today, as we navigate a world of endless feasting, reconnecting with this rhythmic fasting can rejuvenate both body and mind.

Today's frenzied feasting often bewilders our age-old genes. Yet, there's a growing yearning to reconnect with this ancient rhythm—a natural, wintry cadence our bodies once knew so well. The benefits of fasting offer more than just the obvious benefits, like mental space and banishing unwanted weight. It rejuvenates our cells and instills a sense of accomplishment and excitement.

Fasting's Science:

Fat as Fuel: During fasting, our bodies, like a lantern burning through the night, sift through fat reserves, providing a steady, glowing energy. Known as ketosis, this process of burning fat for energy used to happen much more frequently as our eating cycle included more fasting. Our bodies were also much more flexible and able to burn food or our stored fat as fuel as easily as flipping on a light switch. The process of fasting will help reset our ability to flexibly move between fuel sources much more gracefully.

Insulin: Fasting steadies our insulin responses, ensuring a poised metabolic balance. Ensuring our body is responsive to insulin and "listens" to its message is vital to keeping our overall system in peak health.

Our Brain and BDNF: BDNF or brain-derived neurotrophic factor, kindled during fasting, keeps our minds sharp and luminous, brightening our cognitive pathways. BDNF is a small protein produced in the brain that supports the survival of existing neurons and encourages the growth of new neurons. We need this to be able to connect learning and our memory so we can master new skills and store information.

Autophagy: Just as winter prepares the earth for spring's rebirth, fasting rejuvenates us at the cellular level. Ever wondered what happens to damaged or useless cells? Damaged cells don't just disappear on their own. They tend to linger, potentially causing problems if not dealt with properly. This is where autophagy steps in – the cellular process that acts like your body's cleaning crew, breaking down and clearing out those unwanted cells. It's the process where cells break down the damaged junk and reuse the parts. Upcycling at its best! This miracle happens when we quit eating every 4 hours. Autophagy really peaks during a fast between 24 and 48 hours without eating.

Fasting, with its soothing embrace, reduces inflammation, granting us and our digestive tract a peaceful pause. Providing a calm rest to our systems is vital for keeping our body and minds healthy. Breaking a fast is another art form, but really becomes vital if you fast for more than 3 days. Repopulating your digestive tract with helpful bacteria through fermented foods, prebiotics and healthy fats is the key. Making your own fermented foods can be a great new hobby to adopt. Any online search for homemade fermented foods will give you a plethora of new ideas.

Heart Health: To practice fasting is akin to enfolding our heart in a protective, comforting circle. Reducing inflammation and improving the pathways for blood flow, while resetting our appetite is huge for overall well-being. Losing unwanted weight, especially around our midsection is very beneficial.

As we gather our thoughts, bundled up in the knowledge and warmth of fasting's age-old tradition, it's essential to walk this path with mindfulness. This process brings your body renewal and keeping this in mind while banishing thoughts of punishment and lack are the key to success. It's not just about the embrace of winter's chill, but about all the clarity, and cozy moments it can usher in. Before stepping into fasting, remember to consult with your health advisor. As you prepare for your own fasting journey, be prepared for moments of wonder, warmth, and above all, always remember to be kind to yourself.

Chapter 3

The Spectrum of Fasting

Just as winter can range from a delicate flurry to a full-blown snowstorm, fasting, too, has its variations - from gentle pauses to profound breaks. Let's find the method of fasting that best complements your wintry lifestyle - but full disclosure, I use multiple types of fasting every week so I don't believe you will want to focus on only one way. Flexible eating schedules keep our body from getting into a rut. This means the holiday season is the perfect time to begin fasting, as long as our eating schedule isn't 100% yummy treats around the clock . . . balance will be our mantra.

Intermittent Fasting (IF): The Cozy Winter Cabin Approach

Intermittent Fasting (IF) is akin to a cozy winter cabin where you alternate between periods of eating and fasting. Essentially, it involves scheduling your meals within a certain time frame each day, creating a routine that balances nourishment with periods of not eating. This method isn't about what you eat, but rather when you eat, providing your body with regular, predictable fasting periods.

Flavors of Intermittent Fasting (IF):
16/8 Method: The warm tea approach—simple and popular. Enjoy your meals between noon and 8pm, and let the rest be your fasting period. This is one of the most popular forms of intermittent fasting for a reason, it is easy to accomplish for so many people.

Eat-Stop-Eat involves fasting for a full 24 hours, once or twice a week. This method is like a deep, restful pause in your eating routine. By refraining from food for a whole day, you give your body time to rest and rejuvenate. It's a more extended fasting period that may take some getting used to, but it can provide significant health benefits. I encourage you to let your body rest and heal during a 24 hour fast at least two times per week if you can. The process of autophagy is thought to begin around the 17-hour mark of fasting and peaks around 24 hours, allowing this renewal process to happen is so important for long term health.

5:2 Diet: The ever-changing winter week. Eat regularly for 5 days and gently reduce your intake for the other two.

Winter's Tips to Navigate IF's Icy Patches

Snowy Hydration: Remember, water is to fasting as snow is to winter. Essential and pure. Keep your cup filled and sip often.

Gentle Snowfall: When breaking a fast, think of it as the gentle fall of the first snowflake—soft, slow, and deliberate. Sip, bite and chew mindfully and really explore the flavors as they burst on your tongue.

Winter Distractions: Engage in wintry pastimes when hunger nips. Build a snowman, read by the fireside, or take a frosty walk. I find myself to be energetic when fasting and journaling helps me keep my thoughts in order.

Heartwarming Meals: When it's time to eat, choose foods as wholesome as a winter carol.
Nutrient-dense, hearty dishes will fuel your snowy adventures. My absolute favorite this time of year is chia pudding. I take cream, almond milk, chia seeds, cinnamon, walnuts and berries and enjoy my warm flavorful bowl as I break my fast.

IF and The Body's Winter Clock:
Nature knows best. As dusk falls earlier and nights

stretch longer in winter, our bodies too have their circadian rhythm. Embrace IF in harmony with your body's active, awake times, and let fasting coincide with its need for restful, rejuvenating nights. Move your eating window to end earlier when dark falls 3-4 days each week.

Extended Fasting: The Deep Winter Journey
Venturing into longer fasts is like setting forth on a multi-day winter expedition. It's an introspective pilgrimage where the body, like the earth blanketed in snow, takes time to rejuvenate and renew. Each form of fasting offers unique benefits and challenges akin to winter's multifaceted beauty. I highly recommend that you begin with intermittent fasting before jumping into extended fasting. Allow your body to get comfortable with periods of not eating, and become more flexible in using your own body's fat as fuel. Ketosis, the process of burning fat as fuel, needs to become more a way of life before you move into a multi-day fast. This will eliminate the "keto flu" side effects and make fasting a joy rather than a chore.

Utilizing many forms of fasting will keep your body flexible and able to switch between using carbohydrates for fuel as well as ketones for fuel. In the beginning of your journey into fasting, many find their appetite and hunger signals to be quite persistent. Using a variety of approaches will make this process so much easier. Let's explore a few different ways to ease into the warmth of fasting below.

Fat Fasting: The Warm Fire

Fat Fasting can be thought of as a comforting, gradual approach. In this method, you primarily consume high-fat, low-carb foods to encourage your body to enter a state of ketosis, where it burns fat for fuel. This is a less intense form of fasting where you still eat, but you focus on high-fat foods like avocados, and cheese to sustain you.

By limiting protein and carbs, your body is prompted to burn fat for fuel. Over time, this can increase metabolic flexibility, making it easier to switch between carbs and fats as energy sources. Foods allowed on a fat fast include avocados, heavy whipping cream, macadamia nuts, butter, eggs and cheese to name just a few.

To practice Fat Fasting, during your fasting window of 1-5 days, aim for 80-90% of your calories from fats, no sugars and very limited carbohydrates in vegetables. Limit your intake to 1000-1200 calories a day. Think of it as the diet equivalent of a fireplace: limited in scope, but intensely warm.

Bone Broth Fasting: The Comforting Quilt

If fat fasting is the warm fire, bone broth fasting is the plush quilt you wrap around yourself, warding off winter's chill. Bone broth fasting focuses on consuming broth rich in amino acids, collagen, and minerals. According to a study in the 'Journal of Clinical Nutrition', these nutrients are crucial for gut health and tissue repair. Collagen, in particular, has been shown to support joint health and skin elasticity, making bone broth fasting a nutritionally beneficial practice. The amino acid glycine, found abundantly in bone broth, aids in detoxification and can improve sleep quality.

To practice Bone Broth Fasting, during your fasting window of 1-5 days, consume several cups of bone broth. This isn't about starvation but nourishment in a different form. It's akin to switching your winter attire: instead of multiple thin layers, you're donning one thick, snugly coat.

Water-Only: The Untouched Snowfield

Braving a water-only fast is like trekking across a pristine snowfield. Both are challenging yet offer profound clarity. Water fasting prompts the body to enter a deep state of autophagy, where cells conduct a rigorous self-clean-up, removing damaged components. This process is rejuvenating on a cellular level. Moreover, extended water fasts can kickstart ketosis, where the body burns fat reserves for energy. This also leads to the release of ketones, compounds beneficial for brain health.

A Water Fast, as the name suggests, allows you to consume only water—no food. It's straightforward yet can be challenging if you haven't transitioned away from sugar and other carbs. I highly recommend that you try a 2-day fat fast or 2-day bone broth fast prior to beginning water-only fasting. Duration can range from 24 hours to several days, depending on your experience and comfort. Like leaving footprints on an untouched snowy plain, it's essential to move with intention and awareness. Always consult a healthcare professional before embarking on this journey. A hugely helpful tip is to sip "fasting soup" during a water-only fast. Fasting soup is just warm water with salt and pepper added. You can sip this in your favorite mug or eat it with a spoon for that cozy feeling of eating - even when fasting. Stock up on your favorite brewed teas to savor as well. I include my morning cup of coffee on my water-only fasting days as well. I just leave out any cream in my coffee on water-only fasting days. A key to success in water-only fasting is to get your electrolytes.

Fasting Soup Recipe for Success

* Choose a favorite mug or soup bowl.

* Add 1-2 cups of water and heat to desired temperature.
* Add ½ teaspoon of salt. Try a good Himalayan salt or indulge yourself with a smoked salt.
* A few dashes of pepper.
* Enjoy by sipping or savoring with a spoon. After a day of fasting, you will be so amazed by how flavorful and decadent this “fasting soup” tastes.

In the landscape of fasting, there's a method for every type of winter enthusiast. Whether you're seeking the warmth of a gentle fire, the snug embrace of a quilt, or the thrill of untouched snow, fasting offers a variety of experiences, each with its unique allure and benefits. Embrace the season and find your fasting rhythm. Remember the only steadfast rule is to be kind to yourself. If you begin a water-only fast and decide on day 2 that you need some bone broth – have some. You have the rest of your long life to practice different types of beneficial fasts, and let’s be honest with ourselves, a bone broth fast is still leaps and bounds ahead of most holiday eating!

Chapter 4

Seasons and Appetites

As snow settles on rooftops and ice crystals decorate windows, something stirs within us, a longing, an insatiable desire for just one more slice of pie or an extra helping of that creamy soup. Winter, with its charm and challenges, has a profound impact on our appetite. In this cozy corner of our guide, we'll explore why our bellies seem to growl a tad louder as the days grow shorter.

Nature's Influence

Winter's arrival transforms our environment and our daily routines. The shorter days and longer nights don't just prompt us to add more layers to our attire; they also recalibrate our internal clocks. Our circadian rhythms, sensitive to light and darkness, adjust, influencing various physiological processes, including our hunger hormones, ghrelin and leptin. Consequently, our appetite seems as expansive as the winter horizon itself.

Biology of Cold Weather Eating

If you've ever felt an urge to eat just a tad more as the cold sets in, it's not just you—it's biology. Just as squirrels scurry about, collecting nuts for winter, our bodies, too, harbor an ancient inclination to stockpile during the colder months. This isn't just about indulgence; it's survival. Our bodies crave additional calories to generate the heat needed to ward off the winter chill. In essence, every bite is a step towards building a warm, metabolic fire within.

Creamy, winter concoctions that wrap us in a warm embrace from the inside out. Be it a rich stew that's been simmering for hours or a decadent dessert that melts in the mouth; winter is synonymous with comfort foods. But why? Part of it is tradition—those cherished recipes handed down through generations, promising warmth and nostalgia in every bite. But it's also about mood. As the world outside turns gray and frosty, these foods offer a serotonin boost, lifting our spirits and filling us with a sense of well-being. And, of course, with the cold demanding more energy from us, our bodies genuinely need more fuel. So, when you reach for that extra serving, know it's a blend of culture, biology, and sheer winter magic.
Unfortunately, no one told our biology that we don't need extra calories anymore. That is why cozy fasting needs a place in our lives.

Defining Cozy Fasting:
Cozy fasting isn't just about refraining from eating; it's about redefining our relationship with food and winter itself. It's a mindset shift from viewing fasting as deprivation to seeing it as a nurturing practice. This approach integrates health, added time for ourselves, and cozy, comforting activities into a practice that can redefine our winter, overall health, and body. Focusing on delicious warm beverages, flickering candle light and soft, snuggly blankets, we are adding texture to our lives without missing anything necessary. By adopting cozy fasting we are providing the structure our bodies need to navigate winter in a healthy way.

Mindful Munching

It's easy to get lost in the delicious aromas around the holidays. Yet, amidst the whirlwind of feasts and treats, there's a serene space we can retreat to—a space of mindfulness and intentionality. Mindful eating, at its essence, is the act of being fully present during meals. It's about savoring each bite, cherishing every texture, and truly experiencing the culinary wonders winter offers. A combination of fasting periods and mindful eating are the basis of the idea of cozy fasting.

Why Mindful Eating Matters:
By tuning into our meals, we not only enhance the joy

of eating but also develop a deeper connection with our bodies. This heightened awareness helps us recognize true hunger cues, differentiate between physical hunger and emotional cravings, and appreciate the satiety that each meal provides. The result? We relish our winter favorites without going overboard, ensuring that every indulgence is a choice, not a compulsion. If you are feeling a huge hunger pang, go outside and take 10 slow deep breaths. This will help your thinking brain come back on board and allow you to make a conscious decision about your food choice.

Cozy Steps to Embrace Mindful Eating:
Warm Rituals: Begin each meal by taking a deep breath, centering yourself, much like cozying up by a fireplace. Acknowledge the effort, love, and ingredients that went into your dish. This sense of gratefulness will help you truly enjoy the meal.

Savor Slowly: Winter is nature's way of saying, "Slow down." Let your meals echo this rhythm. Chew thoroughly, allowing the flavors to dance in your mouth. You can even choose to put your fork down between bites and take a sip of your beverage.

Plate with Purpose: Use smaller plates or bowls to encourage portion control. The act of refilling can provide a pause, allowing you to check in with your appetite. This trick will allow your brain to feel good about finishing your entire plate.

Distraction-free Dining: Let mealtimes be an escape. Set aside devices, turn off the TV, and immerse yourself in the sensory experience of eating. Let it be as calming as watching snowflakes drift down. Set your table with beautiful dishes, candles and even cloth napkins. Put some mood music on low volume too.

Gratitude and Reflection: End your meals with a moment of gratitude—for the nourishment, the company, and the season. Reflect on your feelings, fullness, and satisfaction. Encourage your family to get involved in making dinner and then be sure and praise the efforts they made.

Impact of Festive Season

When the first snowflake falls, it heralds more than just winter—it announces the beginning of the festive season. From Thanksgiving turkey to Christmas pudding to New Year's champagne, this time of year is a culinary carnival. But beyond the deliciousness, these feasts play into our heightened winter appetite. Families gather, stories are shared, and traditions are celebrated all around the dinner table. This community spirit, combined with the season's natural propensity for indulgence, makes every festive meal feel like a banquet.

In essence, winter's influence on our waistlines is a dance—a dance of biology, tradition, and emotion. As we go through this season, it's essential to understand and embrace this rhythm, finding joy in every bite and every shared meal moment. After all, winter is not just about the cold; it's about the warmth we find in our homes, and our hearts.

As we journey through winter, cozy fasting invites us to redefine our relationship with food and comfort. It's a blend of self-care, mindfulness, and a celebration of life's simple pleasures. By adopting this approach, we not only enhance our health but also enrich our experience of the season, finding joy and coziness in both the foods we eat and the moments we cherish. This mindset shift allows us to approach the New Year with renewed vigor, having embraced a balance that nourishes both body and soul.

Chapter 5

Winter Rhythms

Winter, with its vast white expanse often conjures images of hibernation. Think about the mighty bear, for instance. As it prepares for a long winter's nap, it can consume up to a staggering 90 pounds of food each day. Now, while we aren't bears (and we certainly aren't eating 90 pounds of food per day), there's a parallel in our own behaviors as the cold sets in.

As the chill winds blow, our bodies and minds react to the limited sunlight, often leading to a dip in serotonin levels, that essential feel-good chemical. Our natural response is a gravitation towards carbohydrate-rich comfort foods, like creamy mashed potatoes and freshly baked bread. This is nature's cozy recipe for keeping us content and warm-hearted, even as the world turns into a snowy wonderland.

For some, this seasonal change can lead to Seasonal Affective Disorder (SAD), a more profound mood decline during the colder months. Comfort foods often become a go-to remedy, serving as a culinary balm for the winter blues. While these foods provide temporary solace, it's important to remember that SAD is a condition that may require professional attention. If you're experiencing severe symptoms, consulting with a medical professional is advised. However, for milder cases and the typical winter blues, there are several activities and traditions that can offer relief and joy.

Addressing Seasonal Affective Disorder (SAD)

Recognizing the impact of SAD and the winter blues, it's heartening to know that there are numerous ways to lift our spirits and find comfort during winter's darker days. These remedies and activities, extending beyond the kitchen, provide us with a variety of tools to brighten our days and enrich our experiences.

Here's a cozy guide to navigating the winter blues, blending time-tested remedies with heartwarming activities:

Light Therapy: A bright light box can simulate the serotonin-boosting effects of natural sunlight, tricking the mind into brighter moods.

Aromatherapy: Scents like citrus or lavender can uplift our senses, bringing a slice of summer sunshine into our winter days.

Engaging Activities: Immersing ourselves in hobbies or tasks can be a great distraction from the gloom outside. Whether it's knitting, painting, or puzzle-solving, these activities offer therapeutic benefits.

Mindful Meditations: Grounding ourselves in the moment through meditations, such as a soothing full-body scan, can be a beacon against the shadow of SAD.

Social Connections: Winter might suggest isolation, but it's actually a perfect time to strengthen bonds. Inviting friends over for gingerbread house building or movie nights can be incredibly heartwarming.

By exploring these activities, we not only combat the effects of SAD and the winter blues but also discover new ways to enrich our winter experience. Beyond mere survival, winter becomes a season of thriving, filled with warmth, wellness, and joy.

Beyond the Plate: Nourishing the Soul in Winter
When winter's icy fingers wrap around our world, and the allure of warm, hearty meals grows, it's a delightful opportunity to explore nourishing traditions

beyond just food. The season beckons us to find comfort and connection in ways that satisfy not just our stomachs, but our hearts and souls. Here's a curated list of non-food traditions to infuse warmth into your winter days.

Jolabokaflod (Iceland):
Generally held on Christmas Eve, Jolabokaflod, or the "Christmas Book Flood", is a beloved tradition that began during World War II when foreign imports were limited, but paper was cheap. As a result, books became the gift of choice. On Christmas Eve, Icelanders gift books to each other and then spend the rest of the night reading, often with a cup of cocoa or another warm beverage. Imagine wrapping up a cherished novel, gifting it to a loved one, and then both of you diving into your respective books, the room only interrupted by the turning of pages and occasional sips from a warm drink.

Candlelit Evenings (Scandinavia):
With roots in the Scandinavian concept of 'hygge'—a term that encompasses warmth, coziness, and contentment—candlelit evenings are a way to combat the long, dark winters. As dusk approaches, instead of switching on electric lights, rooms are illuminated with the soft, warm glow of candles. Picture a chilly evening, where the room is bathed in a soft light, shadows dancing on the walls, and there's a tangible sense of calm and coziness.

Nature Crafting (Various Cultures):
Throughout history, humans have used what nature provides for decoration, especially during seasons when resources were scarce. Use winter gifts like pinecones, dried berries, twigs, and fallen leaves to create centerpieces, wreaths, and other decorative items. Crafting a centerpiece for the dining table using pinecones, a few sprigs of holly, and a candle in the middle.

Celebrating the Solstice (Worldwide):
Ancient cultures have long recognized the winter solstice and celebrated it as a time of rebirth, as it marks the shortest day and the return of the sun. Activities can range from lighting bonfires, holding feasts, or quiet reflection. Holding a small gathering, lighting a fire, sharing stories, and celebrating the promise of longer days ahead.

Starry Observations (Global):
Since ancient times, people have looked up at the clear winter skies, observing constellations and seeking meanings in the stars. On a clear winter night, venture out and gaze at the skies. You can even use apps to help identify stars and constellations. Wrapping up in warm blankets, sipping on hot drinks, and watching the Geminids meteor shower in December.

Music and Melodies (Worldwide):
Every culture has its own set of winter or festive melodies that have been passed down through generations. Play or even sing winter-themed tunes that evoke nostalgia and warmth. Gathering around a fireplace, singing carols or playing winter-themed songs on a guitar if you are musically inclined.

Acts of Kindness (Universal):
Acts of giving and kindness are embedded in human culture, more so during times of celebration or hardship. Engage in activities that bring joy to others, be it volunteering, gifting, or simply helping out a neighbor. Organizing a winter clothes drive for the less fortunate or helping an elderly neighbor with their winter chores.

Memory Keeping (Various Cultures):
From scrapbooking in modern times to oral storytelling in ancient cultures, preserving memories has always been cherished. Create a tangible or digital space to store memories, be it photographs, journal entries, or mementos. Crafting a winter scrapbook that captures moments like the first snowfall, family gatherings, and winter adventures.

In our family, we have begun the tradition of painting rocks with holiday themes. Then we leave the rocks at the homes of friends and family and even while out walking to bring joy to those who find them. This year, the kids have created a painted rock advent calendar for my husband and I so we can open a gift each day of December. Then we will decorate our garden with these treasured gifts while saving a few in the storage box with other holiday decorations.

It's easy to get lost in the flurry of cravings and comforts. Another fun activity we practice is to buy a winter-themed puzzle of at least 1,000 pieces and build it together as a family. Learn about traditions of other cultures and ask your friends how they celebrate. Take your favorites and try them this year. With this treasure trove of traditions, we're equipped to embrace the season in all its glory. Cozy fasting, as one more tradition, is not just about saying no to food. It's about saying yes to life's other enriching experiences, wrapping ourselves in warmth, wellness, and intentional living. So as the snow falls and the nights draw in, let's craft a winter that's nourishing in every sense.

Chapter 6

Winter Wellness

As the days shorten and the temperatures drop, the world gets enveloped in a blanket of snow, and everything feels paused, like nature itself is taking a deep breath. However, for some, this seasonal shift isn't just about witnessing the magic of frosty mornings or enjoying the hush of snowfall; it's accompanied by a change in mood, a kind of shadow that dampens the winter wonderland.

The Mystery of SAD

Seasonal Affective Disorder, termed SAD, is more than just "winter blues." It's a type of depression that appears at specific times of the year, most commonly in the fall and continues through the winter months. While everyone might occasionally feel down on a particularly gloomy day, those with SAD experience a consistent and significant change in mood, energy, and behavior.

So, what are the telltale signs? Individuals might experience feelings of hopelessness, lack of energy, changes in sleeping and eating patterns, difficulty concentrating, and even thoughts of self-harm or suicide.

Why Winter, Though?

While SAD can also manifest during spring and summer, its winter occurrence is more common. Several theories try to explain this link between winter and SAD:

Sunlight and Serotonin: Reduced sunlight can lead to a dip in serotonin, a neurotransmitter that influences mood. Lower levels can trigger depression.

Melatonin Matters: The change in season can disrupt our body's internal clock (or circadian rhythm). This can lead to an increase in melatonin production, a hormone responsible for regulating sleep, resulting in feelings of sleepiness and mood changes.

Vitamin D Deficiency: The limited sun exposure during winter can cause a drop in Vitamin D levels, which might play a role in serotonin activity.

Shedding Light on Solutions

Luckily, awareness of SAD has grown over the years, and there's a range of treatments available:

Light Therapy: This involves sitting near a device called a light box, which mimics natural sunlight. This light exposure can cause chemical changes in the brain that lift mood and ease other SAD symptoms.

Medication: Some people with SAD benefit from antidepressant treatment, especially if their symptoms are severe.

Psychotherapy: Cognitive-behavioral therapy can help identify and change negative thought patterns and behaviors that make one feel worse.

Vitamin D: While the direct link between vitamin D deficiency and SAD remains debated, some individuals benefit from vitamin D supplements.

For light therapy, here are the considerations you need to keep in mind when trying this trend out. How do you pick the light box that's your perfect match?

Light boxes for SAD treatment are designed to replicate outdoor light, with the theory that this specific type of illumination can induce a chemical alteration in the brain. This change can help elevate mood and counteract SAD symptoms like excessive sleepiness. But remember, not all light boxes are created equal!

Before You Add to Cart . . .
Before setting your heart on a model, a quick chat with your health care provider can give you clarity. They can guide you on the best light therapy practices tailored for your needs. To make the most of light therapy, generally:

Use the light box within the first waking hour for 20 to 30 minutes.

Place it 16 to 24 inches from your face, but don't stare directly at it.

Opt for a light box that offers 10,000 lux of light but emits as little UV light as possible.

And, since these aren't FDA-regulated specifically for SAD, it's extra crucial to be discerning in your choices.

The Light Box Shopping List
Here's a nifty checklist to consider while scouting for the ideal light box:

Purpose: Is it tailored for SAD treatment? Boxes designed for skin conditions might emit UV light, which can be detrimental to the eyes.

Brightness: Typically, 10,000 lux is recommended. The brighter the box, the less time you'll need to spend in front of it daily.

UV Light Emission: Minimal to zero UV light emission is the goal. Your skin and eyes will thank you.

Eye Safety: Especially if you've got conditions like glaucoma or cataracts, ensure the light box has features to protect your peepers.

Design & Style: From upright lamps to portable rectangular units, choose a style that suits your aesthetic and functional needs.

Positioning: Consider where you'll set it up. Whether you'll be diving into a novel or knitting a scarf, the box should be positioned right for optimal benefits.

Lastly, while some might see them as a luxury, remember that for many, they're an invaluable ally against winter's mental health challenges. So, while it might not be covered by most insurance plans, consider it an investment in your well-being. And again, keep your health care provider in the loop; they might have specific recommendations for you.

Think of a light box as a practical gift you can ask Santa for this Christmas. If you will be purchasing your own, search for: "best light therapy box for treatment of seasonal affective disorder" and then read about the products recommended. Most of the top-rated light boxes are well under $50. Then you can talk to your doctor about your choice to see what they have to say.

Beyond the Traditional – Holistic Approaches

In addition to these remedies, several holistic strategies can complement the healing journey:

Stay Active: Physical activity can help boost serotonin levels and reduce stress, so even a brisk walk outside can be beneficial. My favorite quote is from Vietnamese Buddhist monk, Thich Nhat Hanh, as he says: "When it comes to health and well-being, regular exercise is about as close to a magic potion as you can get."

Stay Connected: Engaging socially can act as a buffer. Whether it's a chat over tea or a snowy walk with a friend, connection matters. Call them on the phone and then begin folding clothes – connection and chores are a beneficial partnership.

Mindful Practices: Techniques like meditation, deep-breathing exercises, and journaling can help in managing stress and increasing self-awareness. Schedule time for this every day to boost the magic.

Establish a Routine: Keeping a regular routine can help counter the effects of disrupted circadian rhythms. Begin each day with a motivating morning routine, read The Shower Habit for some wonderful tips.

Dietary Choices: Eating a balanced diet with mood-boosting foods, like those rich in omega-3 fats, can help counter some of the effects of SAD.

As we navigate winter, with its enchanting beauty and unique challenges, it's essential to be attuned to our well-being. Recognizing the signs of SAD and understanding its seasonal nuances allows us to take proactive steps. In winter, with its extended nights and chilled air, there's an opportunity not just to endure, but to thrive. Through awareness, care, and the right tools, we can turn winter's challenge into an opportunity for wellness, self-reflection, and growth.

Do It Yourself

Painted Snowman Rock Family

Painting rocks is a fun winter activity that can brighten your day. All you need are a few rocks, paint, brushes and some mod podge to seal them. I like to watch fingernail design videos as they are very creative and work on small rocks. Below are instructions for a painted rock snowman family.

Find a rock for each member of your family. Clean them off, let them dry and paint them black. Paint or dab with a q-tip, white paint in three snowman shaped circles. Using a toothpick, dot on eyes and a mouth with black paint. Grab some orange and a toothpick and add the carrot nose.

Get creative with hats and scarves to add personality to each snowman. You can even add team logos to these for unique features. Grab the white and add snow to the bottom for your snowman to rest on. Don't forget the stick arms, or you can draw these on with a lighter colored fine tip sharpie. When it is dry, seal with mod podge. Add these to your inside or outside decor. For a fun twist, you can use your children's fingerprints for the snowman bodies. Get creative and enjoy!

Chapter 7

Beyond the Plate

Winter not only prompts us to seek physical warmth and food, but also to nurture our souls. Fasting when paired with the enchanting beauty of winter is an opportunity to enrich the entirety of our lives. By diving deep into both indoor and outdoor activities that resonate with the season, we can create an ambiance that complements our fasting journey, making it more effective and enjoyable. As we embrace the quiet beauty of winter, let's first turn our attention inward to activities that bolster our emotional health. These practices are not just about passing time; they are gateways to deeper self-awareness and contentment, especially vital during fasting periods.

Emotional Health Activities

Journaling: Documenting your thoughts, emotions, and daily happenings can be therapeutic. It's a space where your words flow uncensored, a haven for self-reflection and understanding.

Crafting: Be it knitting, scrapbooking, or creating handmade gifts, the process of crafting is meditative. Plus, the joy of creating something is incomparable.

Gratitude Rituals: Start or end the day by listing three things you're grateful for. It shifts focus from what's lacking or overwhelming to what's abundant and heartwarming in your life.

Having nurtured our inner selves, it's equally important to engage with the enchanting outdoor world of winter. These physical activities not only invigorate the body but also harmonize beautifully with the fasting process, enhancing its benefits and our overall well-being.

Outdoor Physical Health Activities

Nature Walks:

There's something magical about a winter landscape. Whether it's the pristine snow underfoot, the frozen lakes, or the skeletal beauty of trees, nature walks can be calming. Walking not only aids digestion but also serves as a gentle, grounding exercise during fasting.

Snow Sports:

From skiing and snowboarding to simple sledding or building a snowman, snow sports are exhilarating. They're a great way to stay active, especially if you're on a more relaxed fasting schedule.

Outdoor Meditation:
Find a quiet spot, perhaps in your backyard or a local park. Sit or stand, close your eyes, and take deep breaths. Feel the cold air entering your lungs and the stillness around you. It's a refreshing way to center yourself.

While the winter outdoors offers a unique charm, the comfort of our homes presents another realm of wellness activities. These cozy indoor practices are perfect for days when we seek solace and warmth, complementing the introspective aspect of fasting.

Cozy Indoor Activities
Yoga: Roll out your mat and flow into poses that stretch, strengthen, and relax your body.

Warm Baths: Epsom salts, essential oils, and warm water can create a healing ritual that soothes sore muscles and offers a break from the winter chill.

The joy of winter and fasting can be magnified when shared. Group activities provide a sense of community and connectedness, crucial elements for a fulfilling fasting journey and overall mental health during the colder months.

Group Activities

Group Meditation or Prayer:
Whether you meditate, pray, or do some other form of group reflection, doing it with others can be powerful. It fosters a sense of community and shared purpose.

Discussion Groups/Book Clubs
Form or join a group that discusses books, movies, or even the fasting journey. Sharing experiences and gaining insights from others can be very enlightening.

For instance, consider forming a book club focused on themes of wellness and self-improvement, which resonate with the fasting journey. A great starting point could be Glennon Doyle's 'Untamed', a memoir that explores the journey of self-discovery and the pursuit of a true, untethered life. Its themes of personal growth and breaking free from societal expectations can spark profound discussions, especially relevant for those exploring the transformative experience of fasting. Another excellent choice could be 'Atomic Habits' by James Clear, which delves into the science of habit formation and offers practical advice on making small changes that lead to significant life improvements. Discussing how these insights apply to fasting and overall wellness can provide valuable motivation and camaraderie during the winter months.

After engaging in communal connections, let's not forget the importance of restorative sleep, especially during fasting. The following activities are designed to enhance your sleep quality, ensuring you wake up refreshed and rejuvenated.

Sleep Health Activities

Aromatherapy: Scents like lavender and chamomile can prepare your mind for a peaceful slumber. Use a diffuser in your bedroom or sprinkle a few drops on your pillow.

Digital Detox: Set an hour before bed where screens are off-limits. Instead, read a book, practice deep breathing, or just listen to calming music.

Bedroom Sanctuary: Make your sleep space cozy with soft blankets, blackout curtains, and perhaps even a white noise machine to drown out any disruptive noises.

A well-rested mind is more receptive to activities that further enhance mental clarity and cognitive health. These mental health activities are tailored to complement your fasting journey, offering mental stimulation and peace during the introspective winter season.

Mental Health Activities

Meditation: Even a few minutes of daily meditation can work wonders in clearing your mind and grounding you.

Brain-Boosting Games: Puzzles, board games, or apps that challenge your mind can be both fun and beneficial for cognitive health.

Learning: Winter can be a great time to pick up a new skill or hobby. Online courses, workshops, or simply diving into informative books can stimulate the mind.

Community Service: Winter is an excellent time for outreach. Volunteer at local shelters or organize charity events to strengthen community bonds.

Through this tapestry of activities - emotional, physical, social, and mental - winter becomes more than a season of fasting; it transforms into a holistic journey of wellness. Embracing these practices ensures that our fasting experience is as nourishing for the soul as it is for the body.

Winter, with its unique charm, offers myriad ways to enhance the fasting experience. While fasting might feel like a journey of deprivation at times, combining it with these activities ensures it becomes a holistic experience, nourishing the mind, body, and soul. Your success and contentment with your fasting journey resides in your mindset. Feeling grateful for your health and the new activities that will enrich your life is the way forward.

Chapter 8

Hygge & Fasting + The Challenge

In the heart of Danish homes, there's a secret to beating the winter blues, a cultural gem that has captured imaginations worldwide. It's not just a word; it's a lifestyle, a feeling – it's 'hygge' (pronounced hoo-ga). More than just a word, hygge encapsulates the art of creating intimacy, contentment, and warmth amidst the coldest times. Pair this with the act of fasting, and you've got a potent blend of physical and emotional nourishment.

Historical Roots of Hygge:
Hygge, deeply woven into the tapestry of Danish culture, has become internationally known as the Danish key to happiness. Tracing the origins, some linguistic experts believe the word finds its roots in a Norwegian term for "well-being." And while Norwegians might have coined the word, it was the Danes who truly gave life to its rich, soulful essence.

Denmark, with its prolonged, cold, and dark winters, required not just a physical but also an emotional and psychological survival strategy. The ancient Danes, isolated in their wooden homes amidst the sprawling Nordic landscape, recognized the dire need for warmth — not just against the cold outside but also to fend off the coldness of the soul that the prolonged nights might invite.

Hygge, thus, was an answer to these environmental demands. It wasn't about extravagance but about gratitude — the warmth of a shared meal, the gentle glow of a single candle, the soft embrace of a worn-out quilt. This philosophy is echoed in tales from Denmark's past where the spirit of hygge finds subtle mentions in moments of simplicity, camaraderie, and warmth.

And, as traditions go, they often pass from one generation to the next, each adding their own unique touch. My great-great-grandfather, who emigrated from Denmark, was one such torchbearer of the hygge tradition. Despite the new world he found himself in, he never let go of that intrinsic Danish spirit. Every evening, on his way home, he would buy a bunch of bananas or other fresh fruit delight. It might seem like a simple act, but for him, it was an emblem of joy, a token of togetherness he brought home to his family. This seemingly small gesture created moments of genuine contentment as the family gathered around, sharing stories, laughter, and of course, bananas.

Then there was my grandmother. While bananas became synonymous with joy for her father, for her, it was the daily ritual of a warm bath. She believed in starting her day submerged in warmth. "I just don't feel fresh without having a bath," she would often tell me. And in that act, she found her own version of hygge, a quiet moment of self-care and serenity before the world rushed in.

Through these personal anecdotes and the broader history of Denmark, it becomes clear that hygge isn't merely a word; it's a legacy, a tradition, and a feeling that has been cherished and passed down through the ages.

Hygge Across Cultures:

While the term "hygge" is uniquely Danish, the sentiment it captures is universal. Many cultures, especially those with harsh winters, have evolved their own versions of hygge.

In Sweden, they have "Lagom," which roughly translates to "just the right amount." It's the art of balanced living, of finding satisfaction in moderation. It speaks to a life that's perfectly balanced, not too little, not too much, and resonates deeply with the Swedish ethos.

Norway gives us "Koselig," which, like hygge, pertains to a sense of coziness. Imagine a cold Norwegian evening spent in a mountain cabin with wooden logs crackling in the fireplace, soft candlelight, and a feeling of contentment— that's koselig.

Scotland introduces "Còsagach," inspired by the rugged landscapes and turbulent weather, emphasizing indoor coziness. And then there's the German "Gemütlichkeit" and the Dutch "Gezelligheid," both denoting a sense of belonging, peace, and warmth.

While these terms have their nuances, their essence is strikingly similar— to find warmth, contentment, and joy in life's simple moments. Whether it's the Nordic lands or a remote village in the Alps, people everywhere have always sought and found their unique ways to brave the cold outside by kindling warmth inside.

The Essence of Hygge

Hygge, at its core, isn't about buying a new sweater or sipping a certain type of tea. It's an atmosphere, an experience. Imagine a room lit by only the golden glow of candles, the sound of rain gently tapping on windows, soft laughter shared among close friends – that's hygge. It's simplicity, appreciation, and warmth, distilled into moments.

Nature and hygge are inseparably intertwined. The Danes, like many Nordic cultures, share a deep reverence for the natural world, finding comfort in its rhythms and cycles. Opening your windows each day to replace the air in your home is a part of the hygge experience. In Japan, they call it 'forest bathing' or 'Shinrin-Yoku', but the essence remains universal: immersing oneself in the therapeutic embrace of nature. In Norway they have a saying, “There is no such thing as bad weather, only bad clothes.”

During winter, the skeletal silhouettes of trees against a pewter sky, the hush of snowfall, or the gentle patter of rain against windows can evoke profound feelings of hygge. Even in the heart of bustling cities, these natural moments persist, whispering to us. During your fasting journey, lean into these moments.

Take walks in local parks or gardens, even if it's just a small green patch amidst the concrete jungle.

Create a cozy corner in your home with potted plants, allowing nature to permeate your indoor space.

Listen to natural sounds. The gentle hum of a forest or the soothing lap of waves can be found online and can transport you to a serene place, enhancing the mindfulness that fasting often promotes.

Use natural elements in decor. Think wooden trinkets, pinecones, or a bowl of river stones. Their organic, tactile nature can ground you, invoking the essence of hygge.

Fasting Meets Hygge

Fasting, on the surface, might seem like a stark contrast to the indulgent coziness of hygge. But look a little deeper, and the synergy becomes clear. Both fasting and hygge are about savoring – whether it's the absence of food or the presence of warmth.

Intuitive Eating: Just as hygge teaches us to relish simple moments, fasting can teach us to listen to our bodies, understanding and honoring its signals, and eating not out of habit but genuine need.

Simple Pleasures: In the fasting hours, when the aroma of stew or the sight of a chocolate chip cookie might tempt, we can turn to non-food hygge comforts. A warm bath, a woolen blanket, or a favorite song can be equally satisfying, it's all in our mindset.

Savoring the Break: When it's time to break the fast, make it a hygge moment. Set a beautiful table, light some candles, and enjoy your meal with all your senses.

Hygge-inspired Recipes for Breaking Your Fast:

Breaking a fast deserves a special moment, and what better way to do so than with a dish that's the very essence of hygge - warm, simple, and nurturing.

Hearty Vegetable Stew: Dive into a comforting bowl of warmth with this stew. Start with a base of rich bone broth (or vegetable broth for vegetarians). Add in chunks of cauliflower, zucchini, and bell peppers. Infuse the stew with aromatic herbs like rosemary and thyme. A splash of olive oil and a sprinkle of pumpkin seeds on top bring in richness and a delightful crunch.

Golden Turmeric Tea: This isn't just any tea. It's a blend of warm milk (or a non-dairy alternative like almond milk), a teaspoon of turmeric, a pinch of black pepper, and a dash of honey for those who like it sweet. This soothing drink is not only a hug in a mug but also boasts of the anti-inflammatory properties of turmeric. Perfect for those cool winter evenings!

Creating a Hygge Fasting Environment

Warm Lights: The soft flicker of candles or warm-toned fairy lights can make any space instantly cozier. Whether you're reading, meditating, or just sitting, let this be your backdrop.

Soft Textures: Surround yourself with softness. Think plush cushions, chunky knit blankets, and fuzzy socks.

Engage the Senses: Listen to calming music, burn some incense or essential oils, or indulge in a tactile craft like knitting.

Connect: While fasting can be a deeply personal journey, remember the hygge emphasis on togetherness. Share moments with loved ones, even if it's just a heart-to-heart chat over herbal tea.

Digital Detox and Hygge:
In today's hyper-connected world, our screens often become barriers to genuine moments of hygge. The constant ping of notifications, the unending scroll of social media feeds, and the bright blue light can pull us away from the present moment.

During fasting, when the aim is to connect deeply with oneself, a digital detox can amplify the benefits. Here's why it's crucial:

Mindful Moments: Without digital distractions, we can be wholly present, whether it's savoring a sip of herbal tea, feeling the texture of a woolen blanket, or simply watching the dance of a flickering candle flame.

Deepened Connections: Fasting is as much about introspection as it is about forging deeper bonds with loved ones. Setting the phone aside during meals or intimate moments can lead to richer conversations and shared experiences.

Restful Sleep: If you're fasting during the day, restful sleep at night becomes even more critical. The blue light from our screens interferes with our sleep patterns. Embracing a digital detox, especially during evening hours, can help usher in more restful, rejuvenating sleep.

Incorporating a digital detox during fasting isn't about shunning technology. It's about using it intentionally, ensuring it doesn't overshadow those genuine moments of warmth, coziness, and connection that embody the true spirit of hygge.

The 3 Day Hygge Fasting Challenge

Dive deep into a transformative experience by merging the comforting principles of hygge with the clarifying essence of fasting. Select a fasting method that resonates with you - be it a fat fast, bone broth fast, or traditional water fast. As you proceed, focus on journaling not just your physical sensations but also your emotional journey and reflections inspired by hygge activities.

Day 1: Setting the Scene

Morning: Begin your day with a gentle awakening. Depending on your chosen fast, start with either a bullet-proof coffee or tea with cream (for the fat fast), a warm cup of bone broth, or straight coffee or tea for a water fast. Find a cozy spot, no rush, no devices.

Just you, the morning, and your thoughts. Reflect in your journal about how the morning ritual feels different during fasting. Note any changes in your mental clarity or mood.

Afternoon: Spend some moments in nature. If you're in an urban setting, simply opening a window and listening to natural sounds or having a plant nearby can be a source of connection. Reflect on the calming rhythm of nature and how it mirrors the natural ebb and flow of your hunger and satiety. Record in your journal how this connection to nature influences your fasting experience. Does it enhance your sense of clarity, peace, or introspection? Enjoy "fasting soup" and a cup of tea. Remember to drink plenty of water while fasting.

Evening: Dim the lights, light some candles, and wrap yourself in a plush blanket. As you settle into the night, journal your thoughts about the first day, focusing on the senses awakened by your hygge experiences. Reflect on the important work your body is undertaking. Autophagy peaks around 24 hours into fasting and you are cleaning out damaged cells and rejuvenating your body from the inside out. I love to end the evening with a cup of sleepy-time tea. The delicious tea along with the wishes for a wonderful night of sleep always elevate my mood.

Day 2: Indulging the Senses

Morning: Start with a tactile experience. Feel the textures around you. How does your bed sheet feel? The floor under your feet? As you go about your morning, focus on touch. Drink your morning beverage and savor the flavors.

Afternoon: Listen to calming, soft music, or even better, natural sounds like rain or the rustle of leaves. Let the sounds guide your reflections, especially as you navigate the peak of your fasting period.

Evening: As you prepare for bed, create a spa-like experience in your bath or shower. Pay attention to the smell of your soap and the glide of the loofah on your skin. End your bath with a heated towel and then a self-massage with your favorite moisturizing lotion. Journal your thoughts for the second day of your hygge fast.

Day 3: Deep Reflection and Connection

Morning: Begin your day with meditative practice. Whether it's traditional meditation, a warm bath, or simply sitting with a warm drink. Reflect on the introspective aspect of fasting - how has this journey affected your understanding of hunger, satiety, and self-control? Record these insights.

Afternoon: Connect with someone you cherish – be it a friend, family member, or even a cherished pet. Share a moment of genuine interaction, whether it's a heart-to-heart conversation or a simple shared silence. Buy yourself a book you have been looking forward to and either read or listen to it.

Evening: As you prepare to break your fast, make it a multisensory experience. Notice the colors on your plate, the aroma of your food, and savor each bite.

Before bedtime, light a candle, and reflect on the past three days. As you break your fast, make it a multisensory experience. Note the colors, aromas, and flavors. How does eating feel different now? Write about the joy, gratitude, or any other emotions you experience.

Reflection After the Challenge:

After completing the challenge, set aside time to review your journal entries. Reflect on:

Moments that brought the deepest warmth and comfort.

Changes in your feelings and attitudes towards fasting.

Insights on how integrating hygge enhanced your fasting experience, both physically and emotionally.

This challenge is not just about fasting; it's about discovering a deeper connection with yourself and the world around you through the lens of hygge. Let your journal be a mirror, reflecting your journey and the subtle transformations within.

Chapter 9

Cold Outside, Clean Inside

It's time to reflect on the journey we've undertaken. With each snowflake that descended and each frosty morning we braved, we embraced not just the external cold, but also the cleansing cold within, all thanks to our winter fasting journey.

Winter is nature's way of resetting, shedding the old, and preparing for the new. In sync with nature, our winter fasting has been a detoxifying dance, helping our bodies reset and rejuvenate.

Cellular Renewal through Autophagy:
Fasting activates the body's natural mechanism of autophagy. As we've delved into before, this process cleans out damaged cells, making way for new, healthy ones. In the heart of winter, when nature is seemingly dormant, our bodies have been bustling with regeneration.

Gut Health Restoration:
Winter fasting has given our digestive systems a much-needed break. This rest period can improve gut health, promoting the growth of beneficial bacteria and improving overall digestion.

Boosted Mental Clarity:
Reduced food intake often leads to a sharper mind and increased concentration. This mental detox can be a game-changer, allowing us to welcome spring with a clearer perspective and renewed vision.

Preparing for the Transition into a New Season:
As winter wanes, we begin preparing for the new year. With the clarity winter fasting has brought, it's the perfect time to set intentions for the coming months. What do you wish to achieve? How can you continue the momentum of self-care and mindfulness?

Acknowledge Your Growth:
It's essential to recognize the discipline, resilience, and growth you've demonstrated throughout winter. From navigating holiday festivities with grace to integrating the warmth of hygge, it's been a journey of enrichment.

Consider hosting a "Goodbye Winter" gathering with close friends or family. Reflect on winter memories, share fasting experiences, and toast to the upcoming spring. This event can be not just a farewell to the season but a celebration of the growth and transformation experienced through your fasting journey. Here are some specific suggestions and activities to make your gathering meaningful and memorable:

Theme and Decor:

Embrace a cozy winter theme with soft lighting, candles, and plush throws. Decorate with motifs of snowflakes, pinecones, and evergreens to capture the essence of winter.

Set up a photo corner with winter props and a backdrop of snowy landscapes or a fireplace. This can be a fun spot for guests to take commemorative photos.

Invitations:

Send out personalized invitations, maybe even handcrafted ones, with a note mentioning the significance of the gathering and what guests can look forward to.

Food and Drinks:

Serve a menu of hearty and healthy dishes that align with the fasting journey. Include some of the recipes you've shared in this book, like the Creamy Potato Soup or the Roasted Brussels Sprouts with Brie.

For drinks, offer a variety of herbal teas, warm spiced cider, or even a winter-themed mocktail.

Activities:

Gratitude Circle: Gather around and have each person share something they are grateful for from the past winter. This can be a powerful way to reflect on and acknowledge the season's blessings.

DIY Craft Station: Set up a space where guests can create their own winter-themed crafts, such as painting on stones or assembling small winter terrariums. These can serve as keepsakes to remember the season by.

Recipe Exchange: Invite guests to bring their favorite winter recipe. Set up a recipe exchange corner where everyone can share and take home new ideas for next winter.

Favors:

As a parting gift, consider giving each guest a small token of appreciation, such as a jar of homemade spiced nuts, a scented candle, or a personalized note expressing gratitude for their presence and support.

This 'Goodbye Winter' gathering is more than just a social event; it's a ritual that marks the transition from the introspective winter to the forthcoming vibrancy of spring. It's an opportunity to share, reflect, and set the tone for the months ahead, surrounded by the warmth of friends and family.

By choosing to embark on this winter fasting journey, you've gifted yourself the unparalleled experience of starting the new year riding a wave of accomplishment, rather than being trapped in the quagmire of overindulgence blues.

It's a simple truth, yet profound in its implications: with the right preparation and mindset, fasting can transform from a challenging endeavor into an enriching experience. It's not about deprivation, but about savoring. Savoring those moments of stillness, clarity, and introspection. Moments when the world fades away, leaving only the rhythmic beating of our hearts and the silent dance of snowflakes outside.

And when the fasting window closes, the world bursts into color and flavor again. Because we've granted ourselves this pause, every indulgence becomes more vibrant, every flavor more pronounced. We've learned to indulge on our terms, without the looming dread of side effects, truly savoring each bite, each sip, each laugh shared over a bountiful table.

Carry these lessons with you, not just as memories of a winter gone by, but as guiding stars for the years to come. Let the cozy warmth of hygge, the resilience instilled by fasting, and the jubilant spirit of winter festivities illuminate even the darkest corners, guiding you towards joy, balance, and contentment.

Embrace the seasons ahead with the same zest and zeal, cherishing the warmth you've cultivated from within, and spread it generously, like the first snowfall blanketing the earth. Here's to many more winters of wisdom, wellness, and wonder.

Chapter 10

Recipes to Enjoy and Share

As the days grow colder and the nights stretch longer, our bellies yearn for something scrumptious. How can we indulge in winter's culinary delights while staying aligned with our fasting objectives? The secret: Intentional eating during our eating window and some culinary creativity. Here are recipes tailored for your winter fasting journey, designed to provide comfort without compromising your goals.

Creamy Potato Soup

Embrace the nourishment of a comforting bowl of Creamy Potato Soup, perfect for breaking your fast. Rich in flavor and heartiness, this soup provides the essential nutrients and energy needed after a period of fasting. Its warm, soothing nature makes it an ideal choice to gently wake up your digestive system, ensuring a smooth transition back to regular eating.

Ingredients:

7 medium potatoes, peeled and cubed

1 onion, diced
2 celery stalks sliced
1 garlic clove, minced
1 cup of vegetable broth
3 cup of heavy whipping cream
¼ cup butter
1 cup shredded cheddar cheese
6 slices of bacon cooked and chopped
Salt, pepper, and herbs to taste. I like a pinch white pepper, but the garlic and onions provide great flavor.

Instructions:
In a pot, sauté onions, celery and garlic until soft. Add potatoes, broth, butter and spices, and simmer until potatoes are tender, about 25 minutes. Then add cream, bacon and cheese and cook on low for another 20 minutes.

Roasted Brussel Sprouts with Brie

After a fasting period, it's important to reintroduce foods that are easy on the stomach yet nutrient-rich. These Roasted Brussels Sprouts with Brie are just that. Brussels sprouts are packed with fiber and vitamins, aiding digestion, while the brie adds a touch of indulgence. This dish strikes a balance between health and flavor, making it a delightful way to celebrate the end of your fasting window.

Ingredients:
30 Brussels sprouts cut in half or quarter if large

Olive oil
Salt and Pepper
1 tbsp garlic powder
1/2 tsp red pepper flakes optional
Wedge of brie cheese ~1/3 to 1/2 pound cut into thin slices
1/4 cup pecans roughly chopped

Instructions:
Preheat oven to 400 degrees.
Line a baking sheet with parchment paper.
Place Brussels sprouts in a medium sized bowl and drizzle with olive oil. Add salt and pepper to taste, garlic powder, and red pepper flakes. Toss to combine.
Place Brussels sprouts on baking sheet and bake for 10-15 minutes, until just starting to get soft.
After baking for 10-15 minutes, top with brie cheese and pecans.
Then bake for an additional 10-15 minutes, until cheese is completely melted and just starting to brown.
Serve immediately.

Cinnamon Vanilla Chia Seed Pudding with Walnuts

Chia seeds are a powerhouse of nutrition, and this Cinnamon Vanilla Chia Seed Pudding is a fantastic choice for breaking a fast. The chia seeds provide essential omega-3 fatty acids and fiber, aiding in digestion and gradual energy release. The cinnamon and vanilla offer a comforting flavor, making your first meal back a treat without overwhelming your system. This bowl of goodness can serve as a dessert or a breakfast.

Ingredients:
3 tbsp chia seeds
3/4 cup unsweetened almond milk
¼ cup heavy cream
1 tsp vanilla extract
1/2 tsp cinnamon
A handful of crushed walnuts
Optional: berries or banana

Instructions:
Mix chia seeds, almond milk, cream, vanilla, and cinnamon in a bowl.
Let it sit for a few hours or overnight to thicken. (If you want to add the chia seeds to the almond milk and crush with a spoon, this will speed up the process.)
Top with walnuts and berries before serving. You can even heat in the microwave for 30 seconds if you like it warmed.

Low-Carb Cheesecake

This Low-Carb Cheesecake is a wonderful option for those who want to enjoy without the guilt. The almond flour crust and low-carb sweetener keep it light and digestible, while the cream cheese offers a satisfying richness. It's a perfect example of how a dessert can be both responsible and delicious.

Ingredients:
For the crust:
1 cup almond flour
2 tbsp melted butter
1 tbsp sugar or low-carb sweetener

For the filling:
16 oz cream cheese, softened
1/2 cup sugar or low-carb sweetener
2 eggs
1 tsp vanilla extract

Instructions:
Preheat oven to 325°F.
Mix crust ingredients and press into the bottom of a springform pan. Bake for 10 minutes.
In a bowl, beat the cream cheese and sweetener until smooth. Add eggs one at a time, then mix in vanilla.
Pour the filling over the crust. Bake for 45 minutes or until the center is almost set. Let it cool, then refrigerate for at least 4 hours before serving.

Painted Sugar Cookies

Paint your own sugar cookies before you bake them with this vintage Betty Crocker-Inspired recipe. These are an indulgence!

Ingredients
1 ½ cups powdered sugar
1 cup butter, softened
1 teaspoon vanilla
½ teaspoon almond extract
1 egg
2 ½ cups all-purpose flour
1 teaspoon baking soda
1 teaspoon cream of tartar

Egg Yolk Paint
1 egg yolk
¼ teaspoon water
Food coloring
Food grade paint brushes
Mix these into a small tea cup or paper cup, one for each color.

Steps
In large bowl, mix until creamy: powdered sugar, butter, vanilla, almond extract and egg. Then stir in flour, baking soda and cream of tartar. Cover and refrigerate 2 to 3 hours.

Heat oven to 375°F. Lightly grease cookie sheet with shortening or spray with cooking spray. Divide dough in half. On lightly floured surface, roll each half 3/16 inch thick. Cut into desired shapes with cookie cutters. We enjoy cookie cutters in the following shapes: snowmen, stars, candy canes and reindeer.

On each cookie sheet, place cookies about 2 inches apart. We recommend one cookie sheet for each sugar cookie painter.

In separate small cups, mix 1 egg yolk, ¼ tsp water and food color of your choice. (If paint thickens while standing, stir in a few drops of water.) Paint designs on cookies with small paint brushes. Bake 7 to 8 minutes or until edges are light brown. Remove from cookie sheet to wire rack; cool.

Let these dishes be your culinary companions during winter, ensuring that every bite aligns with the rhythm of your fasting journey and the coziness of the season. Cheers to delightful dishes and mindful munching!

Chapter 11

Cozy Gift Ideas

Many of these ideas have been listed previously, but this is the one-stop-shop for your convenience. Giving gifts to friends and loved ones can be a cherished task or a stress-inducing, budget-busting, sugar-laden whirlwind. Stress can detract from the true meaning and joy inherent in the act of giving. Incorporating mindfulness into your approach can greatly alleviate these anxieties, allowing for more deliberate and thoughtful decisions. Let's explore some carefully curated ideas designed to stimulate your creativity and elevate your gift-giving strategy this holiday season.

Here are a few homemade gifts that will delight your friends and family.

Homemade Gifts: Crafted with Love
Salt Dough Ornaments
A classic and heartfelt way to add a personal touch to your tree or gift a cherished memory.

Ingredients:
2 cups all-purpose flour
1 cup salt
1 cup water

Instructions:
Mix ingredients to form a dough.
Roll out and shape using festive cookie cutters.
Create a small hole for hanging.
Bake at 250°F for 2-3 hours or until completely dry.
Once cooled, paint and decorate!

Choosing simple shapes, adding twine and drawing details with fine tip sharpies can be beautiful.

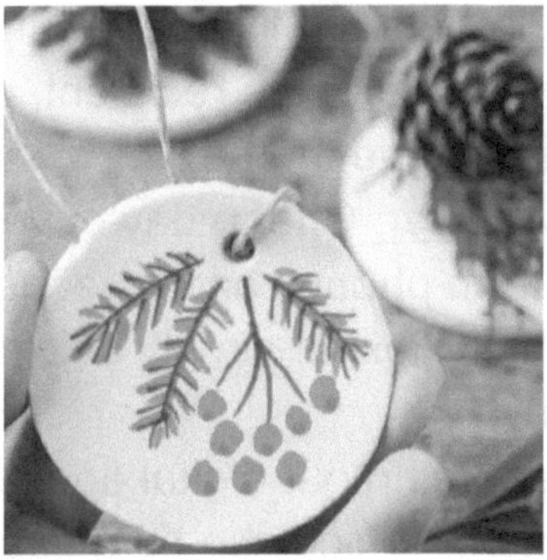

Spiced Nuts
An aromatic blend that promises a burst of flavor in every bite, perfect for gifting.

Ingredients:

2 cups raw cashews, walnuts or pecans
1 tbsp melted butter
2 tsp cinnamon
1 tsp ground ginger
Pinch of clove
Salt to taste

Instructions:
Mix ingredients and spread out on a baking sheet. Bake at 300°F for 15-20 minutes or until toasted. Let cool and pack into decorative jars.

Nature Crafting: Collect pinecones, twigs, and other treasures from nature. Craft them into wreaths, centerpieces, or ornaments.

Personalized Playlists or Mixtapes: Curate a list of songs that remind you of the recipient, or songs that fit the winter and hygge theme.

Digital Detox Voucher: Offer a day of your undivided attention, free from phones and screens. It can be a day of shared activities, or simply enjoying each other's company.

Handwritten Letters: In our digital age, a personal, handwritten note or recipe can be a heartwarming gift. Share fond memories, express gratitude, or simply recount the highlights of the past year.

Experience Gifts: Memory Makers

Instead of the usual material gifts, consider gifting experiences that foster connection and lasting memories:
* A pottery class, where you both can craft something beautiful.
* A dinner cruise or guided tour of a local landmark.
* A cozy stay-at-home movie night kit, complete with a soft blanket, classic holiday films, and gourmet popcorn.
* A visit to a local winter festival or holiday light display.

Hygge Enhancers: Shop with Intention

For those seeking tangible gifts, consider items that boost the hygge vibes:
* Scented Candles: Opt for festive scents like pine, cinnamon, or cranberry.
* Chunky Knit Blankets: Nothing spells cozy better.
* Tea Sets or Gourmet Hot Cocoa Kits: Warm drinks for chilly nights.
* Cozy Slipper Socks: Footwear fit for a hygge champion.
* Aromatherapy Kits: Essential oils like lavender, chamomile, or eucalyptus can help in relaxation and enhancing the overall hygge experience.
* Ceramic Mugs: For those warm drinks on cold nights, a beautiful mug can make each sip feel even more special.
* Light Box: Use for Seasonal Affective Disorder light therapy and a serotonin boost.

Festive Family Traditions: Building Bonds

Holiday Puzzles:

Make it an annual affair to work on a holiday-themed puzzle together. It's not just about the end picture, but the stories and conversations shared piece by piece.

Customized Advent Calendars:

Invest in a beautifully crafted wooden advent calendar with little numbered drawers. Each year, fill it up with tiny trinkets, notes, or even challenge prompts (like "sing a carol" or "write a gratitude note"). It's a gift that grows with memories and traditions.

A New-to-you Board Game

There are so many new family board games to play! Maybe you are good at the tried-and-true Monopoly and Sorry, but you need to check out the many versions of Clue and we love Sequence and Blokus.

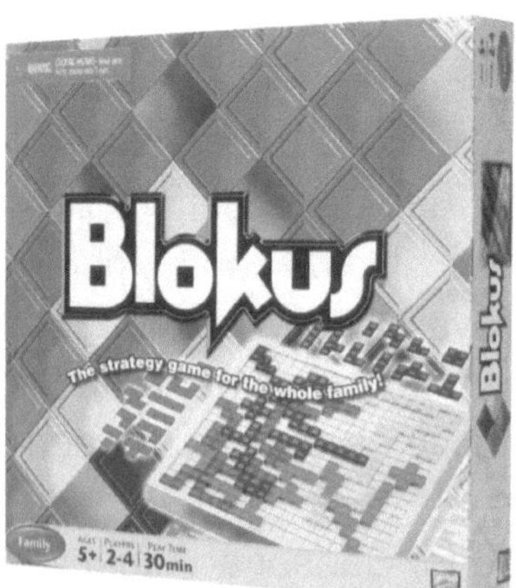

The holidays can often feel like they're pulling us in a hundred different directions. By grounding our actions in intention and a genuine desire for connection, we can transform this season from one of stress and consumption to one of joy, mindfulness, and authentic celebration.

Each gift, regardless of its cost, carries the essence of thoughtfulness, warmth, and the spirit of hygge. Remember, it's the intention and love behind the gift that truly counts.

Find many more short, supportive books to enhance your journey to health and happiness at https://stephanieewingauthor.com and follow Stephanie on Amazon to learn about new releases and book discounts.

Resource:

Fasting Protocols

As you're savoring this cozy fasting book, you've probably come to realize that fasting comes in many shapes and sizes, much like your grandma's patchwork quilt. We've all got our unique tastes, health goals, and holiday traditions—so why should our fasting approach be any different? A season of cozy blankets, warm fires, and… fasting?

Absolutely, you can do this, get healthier, be merry and above all, be kind to yourself. Give yourself grace and find the tips that work for you. You can enjoy the holidays and stay on track with fasting. Whether you're contemplating drizzling some heavy cream into your coffee or sipping bone broth like it's your grandma's secret recipe, this chapter is where you'll find your comfy match.

How to Fat Fast: A Practical Guide
Listen to your body. Eat when you're hungry, and continue eating until you feel satisfied. There's no need to rigidly schedule your meals – let your hunger guide you.

Foods to Embrace:

Feel free to add up to 3 tablespoons of heavy cream to your tea or coffee.
Eggs: Boiled, fried in healthy oils, or scrambled with ghee.
Bacon: Opt for those without added sugars or harmful additives.
Fatty Fish: Salmon and sardines are particularly rich in beneficial fats.
Oils: Olive oil, coconut oil, MCT oil, avocado oil, and macadamia nut oil.
Solid Fats: Butter and ghee are both excellent sources of healthy fats. Make sure they are high-quality and, when possible, organic.
Mayo: Make sure it's made from a healthy oil base, without added sugars or unhealthy additives.
Avocado: In slices, as a salad, or even as a guacamole (minus the dairy).
Olives: They're a great snack, and they're packed with healthy fats.
Leafy Greens: They're excellent when cooked in oils or fats, like a spinach sautéed in coconut oil or a kale salad drizzled with olive oil.
Spices: Feel free to season your foods! Just be cautious of spice blends that might contain sugars or additives.

Drinks:
Bone Broth: It's hydrating and packed with minerals, making it perfect for fasting. Opt for high-quality, organic varieties.

Tea/Coffee: Both can be consumed, but keep an eye on caffeine intake and avoid adding sugars.
Bubbly Water: Infused with natural flavor, no calories.

Challenge/Misconception: Many people believe that consuming high-fat foods during a fat fast will lead to weight gain or health issues.
Clarification/Solution: It's important to understand that a fat fast is designed for short-term use, primarily to break through weight loss plateaus or jumpstart ketosis. The high intake of healthy fats can actually help to satiate hunger and stabilize blood sugar levels. It's critical, however, to focus on healthy fat sources like avocados, nuts, and olive oil, and to remember that this approach is not intended for long-term dietary habits.

Challenge/Misconception: There's a misconception that you can eat unlimited amounts of fat during this fast.
Clarification/Solution: Portion control is still key in a fat fast. Even though the focus is on healthy fats, consuming them in moderation is essential to avoid overconsumption of calories. Paying attention to your body's hunger cues and stopping when you feel satisfied is crucial.

Fat fasting offers a streamlined approach to intermittent fasting, focusing heavily on healthy fats. By simplifying your dietary choices, you can enhance the benefits of fasting, all while relishing in tasty foods that keep you satiated. Remember, the fat fast isn't a long-term solution but a tool to break plateaus or jumpstart ketosis. Always consult with a health professional before making significant changes to your diet.

How to Bone Broth Fast: A Practical Guide

Trust your instincts and drink bone broth whenever you feel hungry. It's about listening to your body and addressing your hunger cues without solid food.

Bone broth fasts typically last 24-72 hours. It's essential to choose a duration that feels right for you and to consider consulting with a health professional. Opt for high-quality, organic bone broths, preferably homemade or from trusted suppliers. This ensures you're getting the maximum nutrient value without unwanted additives.

Types of Bone Broth:
Beef: Made using beef bones, rich in collagen, and has a robust flavor.
Chicken: Offers a lighter taste and is packed with essential nutrients.
Fish: A good source of iodine and omega-3 fatty acids.
Nutritional Value: Bone broth is filled with minerals (like magnesium, calcium, and phosphorus), amino

acids, and collagen, all beneficial for gut health, joint health, and overall well-being.
Herbs and Spices: Feel free to infuse your bone broth with herbs like rosemary, thyme, or turmeric for added flavor and health benefits. Ensure that any spices you use do not contain additives or sugars.
Vinegar: A splash of apple cider vinegar can help extract more minerals from the bones.

Challenge/Misconception: Some individuals believe that bone broth fasting doesn't provide enough nutrients and may lead to nutrient deficiencies.
Clarification/Solution: While bone broth is not as nutrient-dense as whole foods, it is rich in minerals and amino acids that support gut health and joint function. This type of fast is generally safe for short periods (24-72 hours). If you plan to extend the duration, it's advisable to consult a healthcare professional and consider supplementing with vitamins and minerals.

Challenge/Misconception: There's a concern that bone broth fasts are not filling, leading to extreme hunger.
Clarification/Solution: Bone broth is surprisingly satiating due to its high protein content. If hunger becomes a challenge, consider increasing the frequency of broth consumption or incorporating a small amount of solid food, such as steamed vegetables, into the fast.

Remember to drink enough water. You can also enjoy tea, and coffee. Bone broth fasting offers a nourishing approach to intermittent fasting, providing the body with essential nutrients while allowing the digestive system to rest. It's an age-old remedy that combines the benefits of prolonged fasting with the nourishment of bone broth. But, as with all dietary changes, it's essential to ensure it's right for your individual health needs. Always consider seeking advice from a health professional before embarking on a bone broth fast.

How to Water Fast: A Comprehensive Guide

Water fasting means consuming water when you feel thirsty. Always prioritize your body's signals and ensure you're staying adequately hydrated.

The length of a water-only fast can vary, from 24 hours to several days. If you're new to fasting, consider starting with shorter durations and gradually increasing as you become more accustomed. Always consult with a healthcare professional before attempting longer fasts.

Water Quality: Aim for pure, filtered water. You may want to avoid tap water that may contain contaminants or added chemicals, although I enjoy my well water when fasting. Spring water or mineral water can also be good choices. Water fasting can potentially help the body with detoxification, promote autophagy (a cellular cleanup process), and offer a mental clarity that some fasters report.

Your meal plan for this fast is water, water and more water. No broths. Just pure H2O. Herbal teas and coffee can complement your fast. Try Fasting Soup which is just warm water with added salt and pepper.

Precautions:
Stay Hydrated: While it's a water fast, it's essential not to over-hydrate. Drink when thirsty.
Monitor Physical Activity: During a water-only fast, your energy levels might differ from the norm. It's recommended to avoid strenuous activities.
Break the Fast Carefully: When coming out of the fast, especially if it's extended, reintroduce foods slowly. Start with light, easily digestible foods.
Seek Medical Advice: Especially important for those on medication, with medical conditions, or attempting longer fasts. Always consult with a healthcare professional to ensure safety.

Challenge/Misconception: A common misconception about water fasting is that it's a quick fix for rapid weight loss.
Clarification/Solution: Water fasting should not be approached as a quick weight loss solution. It's a more intense form of fasting that requires proper preparation and mindset. The weight loss on a water fast can be significant, but it's vital to transition back to normal eating patterns carefully to maintain health and avoid rapid weight regain.

Challenge/Misconception: There's a belief that exercising during a water fast boosts fat loss. Clarification/Solution: During a water fast, the body's energy levels can vary. Strenuous exercise is not recommended as it can lead to fatigue and dizziness. Light activities like walking or gentle yoga are more suitable. Always listen to your body and rest when needed.

Water-only fasting is a profound experience and a journey of self-discovery for many. It offers a reset for both the body and mind. However, safety should always be the utmost priority. Listening to one's body, being aware of one's limits, and seeking professional advice can make the process both beneficial and enlightening.

Importance of Hydration, Electrolytes, and Supplements While Fasting

Fasting, when done with intention and care, can be a rejuvenating experience for the mind and body. When done correctly and safely, fasting can actually improve metabolic health. It's important to ease into fasting, especially if you're new to it, and to always listen to your body. Starting with shorter fasting periods and gradually increasing them can help your body adapt more comfortably. It's also essential to recognize that as we abstain from food, the body's usual sources of essential nutrients and water diminish. This makes hydration, electrolytes, and, in some cases, supplements, of paramount importance.

Water plays a vital role in every cell and function in our body, from waste removal to temperature regulation. As the body taps into fat stores for energy, it releases toxins. Water helps flush these out. Another tip to remember, since we get a significant amount of our daily water intake from food, fasting can increase the risk of dehydration.

Getting your electrolytes when fasting can be an overlooked element. Electrolytes are minerals that carry an electric charge, critical for many bodily functions. Electrolytes like potassium and magnesium prevent muscle cramps and weakness. Sodium, calcium, and potassium are essential for transmitting electrical signals in the nervous system.

Remembering your electrolytes can help prevent "Refeeding Syndrome". This can occur when reintroducing food after prolonged, multi-day fasting. Ensuring you have adequate electrolytes during the fast can mitigate this risk.

While short fasts might not require any additional supplementation other than added salt in your water periodically, longer fasts can deplete certain essential nutrients.

Vitamins: Water-soluble vitamins, like vitamin C and the B vitamins, are not stored in significant amounts in the body and can be depleted during longer fasts.
Minerals: Calcium, potassium, magnesium, and zinc are crucial for numerous biochemical reactions in the body.
Fatty Acids: Especially if you're on a prolonged fast, essential fatty acids might be needed.
Fiber: While not a supplement in the traditional sense, some individuals opt for a soluble fiber supplement during longer fasts to support digestive health.

The need for hydration, electrolytes, and supplements can vary based on whether you're on a complete fast, water fast, bone broth fast, or any other type of restricted caloric intake. Always consult with a healthcare professional to determine your unique supplementation needs.

Fasting FAQs

Is fasting safe? For most people, fasting is safe and can even be beneficial. However, always consult with a healthcare professional before starting, especially if you have underlying health conditions or are on medication.

Will I lose muscle mass during fasting? Not typically. Short-term fasts have been shown to preserve muscle mass, and your body first uses glycogen and fat for energy before tapping into muscle.

Can I drink water during a water-only fast? Absolutely! In fact, staying hydrated is crucial. You can also drink non-caloric beverages like black coffee or tea.

I'm diabetic. Can I fast? If you're diabetic, especially if you're on medication, it's essential to consult with your doctor before starting any fasting regimen. I would also highly recommend you read The Diabetes Code by Dr. Jason Fung.

Will I be constantly hungry while fasting? Not necessarily. While you might experience hunger pangs initially, many people find they diminish over time. Plus, the body starts producing more of the hormone ghrelin, which can actually make you feel full.

How can I manage hunger during fasting? Drink plenty of water, stay busy, and remember, herbal tea or bone broth (in certain fasts) can be a lifesaver. Also, hunger comes in waves; it'll pass! You can try "fasting soup" which is just salt and pepper in warm water. Or you can use a crutch and drink bone broth. Many will tell you that this is "breaking" your fast and yes, it technically does. But fasting is a journey and bone broth allows you to fast - then you do you!

Can I exercise during a fast? Yes, but listen to your body. Light to moderate exercise can be done, but maybe save the high-intensity workouts for non-fasting days or after you've broken your fast.

How often should I fast? It depends on your goals and how your body responds. Some people do intermittent fasting daily, while others do extended fasts less frequently.

Can I take medications while fasting? Always consult with your doctor regarding medications and fasting. Some medications need to be taken with food.

Will fasting slow down my metabolism? No. Short-term fasting has been shown to increase metabolic rate slightly. However, very long-term fasting (beyond 72 hours) might have a different effect.

I didn't reach my fasting goal. What now? That's okay! Every hour you've fasted still provides benefits. Take note of how you felt, adjust if needed, and try again. Fasting is a journey, and every step counts.

Can pregnant or breastfeeding women fast? Fasting is generally not recommended for pregnant or breastfeeding women. Always prioritize the health and nutritional needs of both mother and child.

Remember, fasting is as much an act of nourishing as it is an act of abstaining. By ensuring you're well-hydrated, replenished with essential electrolytes, and supplemented when needed, you're setting the stage for a beneficial and healthful fasting experience. Always listen to your body's signals, and when in doubt, seek guidance. After all, fasting is a journey, and every step should be taken with care and mindfulness.

Resource:

Fasting Around the World

The concept of fasting, especially during winter, isn't confined to a specific region or culture. It's a practice that spans continents, driven by a blend of tradition, religion, and sometimes, sheer necessity. Let's embark on a global journey to understand how different parts of our world embrace fasting amidst the chill of winter.

Scandinavia: Fasting & Festivity
In the land of the Northern Lights, fasting isn't particularly a winter routine. However, Scandinavia is no stranger to the concept. Historically, limited food supply during harsh winters would naturally lead to periods of reduced intake. Today, however, the fasting spirit can be seen in their deep appreciation for 'hygge,' which emphasizes comfort, connection, and moderation.

Russia: The Nativity Fast
Winter in Russia is synonymous with the Nativity Fast, a religious period leading up to the Orthodox Christmas. Spanning 40 days from November to January, it's a time when meat, dairy, and eggs

traditionally don't grace the dinner table. However, fish, vegetable stews, and grains become staple foods.

India: The Karva Chauth & Other Fasts

While India is a land of diverse cultures and an array of festivals, winter is marked by specific fasting rituals. One notable fast is 'Karva Chauth,' where married women fast from sunrise to moonrise for their husbands' longevity. Warm, spiced teas and hearty porridges break the fast.

Middle East: Winter & Religious Reflection

While the well-known Ramadan doesn't fall in winter, several other minor fasting days in Islamic tradition might. These fasting days, like the Day of Ashura, involve refraining from food and drink from dawn until sunset, with evenings celebrated with dates, warm broths, and communal prayers.

Japan: Fasting & Zen Buddhism

In the tranquil temples of Japan, monks often engage in intermittent fasting as a spiritual practice. Winter, with its reflective mood, is a perfect time for this. The idea is not just about abstention but also about mindfulness and gratitude for whatever little is consumed, often in the form of warm broths and teas.

Native American Tribes: Fasting & Vision Quests

For many indigenous tribes in North America, fasting was sometimes part of winter vision quests—spiritual rituals to gain insight or direction. These fasts were not just about food but also about solitude, introspection, and connecting with nature's rhythms.

Fasting, in its many forms across the globe, is often less about the act itself and more about the deeper intentions behind it—whether spiritual, communal, or personal. Winter, with its introspective ambiance, naturally complements these fasting traditions. As we embrace cozy fasting, it's heartening to remember that we're part of a global tapestry, each thread woven with tales of resilience, reflection, and rejuvenation.

Do It Yourself

Christmas Book Flood

Planning your own family Christmas Book Flood, or Jolabokaflod, can be an enchanting tradition that combines the love of reading with the joy of the holiday season. To make this experience truly memorable, let's delve into creating a cozy atmosphere and explore a sample list of books with brief descriptions to help you choose the perfect reads for your loved ones.

Creating a Cozy Atmosphere:

Reading Nook: Set up a comfortable reading nook in your home with soft pillows, warm blankets, and gentle lighting. Add a string of fairy lights for a magical touch.

Snacks and Drinks: Prepare some comforting winter snacks like gingerbread cookies or cinnamon rolls. For drinks, hot cocoa, spiced cider, or herbal teas make perfect companions to a good book.

Background Music: Play some soft, instrumental music in the background to enhance the ambiance. Classical, jazz, or acoustic tunes can be excellent choices.

Book Recommendations with Descriptions:

Adult:

Lessons in Chemistry by Bonnie Garmus: This novel, set in the 1960s, follows the extraordinary life of chemist Elizabeth Zott, whose unconventional approach to life and love challenges the societal norms of her time.

The Bucket List by Rachel Hanna: A heartwarming story about discovering life's possibilities, following a character who embarks on an adventure to complete a bucket list, after her friend requires it in her will.

The Curious Incident of the Dog in the Night-Time by Mark Haddon: Told from the perspective of a 15-year-old boy with autism, this mystery novel is a captivating journey through a unique mind, filled with unexpected twists and emotional depth.

The Checklist Manifesto: How to Get Things Done Right by Atul Gawande: A non-fiction book that explores the idea of using checklists in complex processes, offering insightful and practical approaches to problem-solving and efficiency.

Nom Nom Paleo: Food for Humans by Michelle Tam and Henry Fong: Perfect for food lovers, this cookbook is a delightful blend of humor, stunning photography, and delicious paleo recipes.

Picture Books:

The Book With No Pictures by BJ Novak: A playful and imaginative book that proves words alone can be fun and engaging, encouraging children to explore the power of language.

The Dot by Peter H. Reynolds: A beautifully illustrated story that inspires creativity and confidence by showing how a simple dot on a page can lead to a journey of self-expression and discovery.

The Invisible String by Patrice Karst and Joanne Lew-Vriethoff: This heartwarming book explores the invisible connections of love and reassurance that bind us, perfect for children dealing with separation anxiety or loss.

With these cozy setup ideas and your hand-picked selection of books, your Christmas Book Flood can be an unforgettable tradition that nurtures the love for reading and creates cherished holiday memories.

Thank you for reading Cozy Fasting: Healthy & Hygge Habits During the Holiday Season. I love to hear from readers so please reach out if you have comments! If you have a moment, please leave a review or click the stars at the end of the ebook. It really helps!

About the Author

Stephanie Ewing is a bestselling author in the field of personal development. Her work can be explored in greater depth at www.StephanieEwingAuthor.com, where numerous FREE resources await. Stephanie's approach is characterized by honesty, humor, and practicality. She tackles topics she believes are pivotal to achieving happiness, such as developing energizing habits, managing anxiety, boosting confidence, and enhancing overall health.

Her books are inspired by a career rich in learning and diverse life experiences, reinforcing her belief that true strength emanates from within. Among her notable works are 'The Shower Habit', 'The Sleep Habit', and 'The Fasting Habit', each based on the principle of small, impactful habit changes leading to significant life improvements.

A particularly touching and unique addition to her book list is 'When Boobs Attack', a memoir co-authored with a friend who, alongside Stephanie, battled breast cancer. This book is written with candor and wit, offering an insightful and often humorous perspective on a journey through illness and recovery.

Stephanie's academic journey began with business administration and marketing, eventually pivoting to a fulfilling career in public education. Her two decades of leadership in this field, coupled with a passion for behavior change, fueled her transition to becoming a writer.

When not on her mission to enhance lives through simple habit transformations, Stephanie is an avid reader, podcast enthusiast, vacation planner, and nature walker. She resides in the Pacific Northwest with her family and a small menagerie of farm animals, where the rolling farmlands continually inspire her writing and personal growth.

**For a peek at The Shower Habit: 10 Steps to Increase Energy, Boost Confidence and Achieve Your Goals Without Waking Up Earlier, keep reading!

The Premise & Quiz

The Shower Habit will teach you how to:

- start your day with confidence without getting up earlier,

- boost your productivity in meeting your goals,
- reduce stress, and
- increase happiness.

All by following this simple morning habit. Don't miss this opportunity to make over your morning routine, motivating you to take action toward your goals. These simple changes will transform your life!

You're busy. I get it. You work. You have a family, friends, a pet (or few). It is a lot without adding anything else to your plate, but let me ask you this: Is your current reality exactly where you want to be?

Do you dream of a vacation to the Caribbean?

Do you want to write a book?

Do you want to run a marathon or learn to play the piano?

Whatever your dreams are, you owe it to yourself to try this. You deserve it. After incorporating the Shower Habit into your day, you will have the motivation to take action to achieve your goals. Increased energy and happiness levels will do wonders for your ability to finish the tasks that lead to your desired outcomes. You are not lazy. You are not a hopeless procrastinator. You just need to practice a little self-care by ramping up your morning routine. This process is designed to be enjoyable, rewarding, and highly addictive, so you won't want to miss it!

Let's begin by assessing your shower. Take this quiz to determine if you need to stop reading and make environmental changes or if you score high enough to keep reading.

Shower Quiz

Each question is worth 1 point:

1. Is the bathroom where you shower clean?
2. Does your bathroom have a pleasing scent?
3. Do you have a device in your bathroom that allows you to play music?
4. Do you have a nice, soft towel?
5. Do you have a mirror in your bathroom?
6. Do you have a clock or timer in your bathroom?

If you scored 5–6 points, you are ready to keep reading!

If you scored 3–4 points, you could keep reading, but you may want to consider making changes to your bathroom first.

If you scored 2 or below, stop reading and go make some changes to your bathroom. When your bathroom space can score at least a 3 on the above quiz, then you are ready to keep reading.

Bathroom Makeover

If you scored low on the quiz, I want to help you have the best space possible to complete your Shower Habit. First, let's take it to a basic level of cleanliness. Sweep and mop the floor, wipe down the counter, and clean the mirror. Take a toilet brush to the toilet and wipe off the back of the toilet. Find or buy a candle or something that smells good for the back of the toilet. Now, you can add two points for clean and smells good.

Next, add a clock or digital timer to your bathroom. You must be able to see it from your shower. I guess, if your phone is waterproof, you can take that in, but I really don't recommend that. Phones are too distracting. You can leave your phone on the counter and play some music AFTER you step out of the shower. Now, you can add two more points to your quiz for music and clock.

Finally, the last touches to be extremely ready for your morning routine are a soft, clean, great-smelling towel and a mirror. If you live in a shared bathroom situation, grab a bathroom caddy and put all of your goodies into it—soft towel, mirror, phone, Clorox cleaning wipes, soap, shampoo, lotion, something that smells good, and a dry erase marker.

You have now scored 100 percent on the quiz and are ready to kick some Shower Habit booty!

Made in United States
Troutdale, OR
07/10/2024

21139814R00066